April 2010

THEATRE AND THE MIND

To Dean,

with all best wishes,

Mick.

Mick Gordon

Theatre and the Mind

OBERON BOOKS
LONDON

First published in 2010 by Oberon Books Ltd
521 Caledonian Road, London N7 9RH
Tel: 020 7607 3637 / Fax: 020 7607 3629
e-mail: info@oberonbooks.com
www.oberonbooks.com

A catalogue record for this book is available from the British Library.

ISBN: 978-1-84002-876-8

Printed in Great Britain by CPI Antony Rowe, Chippenham

Contents

Introduction

I'M IN A theatre. The lights go down. Silence. I'm in the dark. Nothing. I hear music. Information. Some lights illuminate. Information. I see a portion of an obviously artificial setting. Information. A person enters; an actor. He is going to pretend to be someone that he is not. I do not think this strange, I do not think at all. I search his face. Information. He is wearing a costume. Information. He walks in a certain way. Information. I watch and listen. Then the actor speaks.

All theatre happens in the mind. What occurs on the stage is a contrivance, an illusion, presenting us, the audience, with specifically chosen information. The quality of that information and how it is communicated will vary, but regardless of quality, when we are in the theatre our minds suspend their disbelief and legitimise the illusion. And it is our minds that pull the experience of theatre together with a single silent question: 'What's the story?'

Again the lights go down. Silence. I'm in the dark. Nothing. I hear music. The radio? Yes, it's the radio. I'm in a bed. It must be my bed. I open my eyes. I see a portion of a room. A bedroom. It's my bedroom. A person enters; a woman. It's my wife. I do not think this strange, I do not think at all. I search her face. She's preoccupied. No. She's pissed off. She is wearing some clothes but not fully dressed. Ah! A fashion crisis. She walks in a certain way. Quickly. She's tense. I watch and listen. And then she speaks.

All life does not happen in the mind. But it is our minds that consciously experience and explain all life. And as I wake from a dreamless sleep it is my mind that pulls my life together, with the same silent question: 'What's the story?'

Minds are what brains do. They are brains in action. The brain evolved as a means of orchestrating adaptive interaction between the organism – us – and the physical and social world. The mind is the product of that interaction. The most important biological function of the brain is to generate behaviours, which is to say, actions that promote the welfare of the organism. In situations of rest or emergency the brain instructs reflex action. When not in situations of rest or emergency the brain has time for consciousness. These are the moments when we experience ourselves as *our selves*.

Our minds make us up. It is our minds that consciously experience our emotions, thoughts and actions. And it is our minds that consciously consider our future emotions, thoughts and actions. Our idea of our self, of what it means to be a person and indeed what is means to be a certain type of person, is therefore dependent on our mind. They are our storyteller, rationalizing and editing explanations for our feelings, thoughts and behaviours, settling on the story that seems most plausible, and offering imagined future scenarios based on that story. And so we conclude that we have made choices. And this is why we believe we have free will.

But consciousness and the stories our minds are telling us happen after the fact. Action, emotion and thought happen first. Consciousness and its accompanying story happen second. I find myself walking outside and putting a cigarette in my mouth. As I'm about to light it: 'What's the story?' 'You want a cigarette.' Our minds tells us stories that justify our actions, thoughts and feelings before giving us access to choice or to alternative points of view. This is why in an argument most of us believe our opening position to be the reasonable one. In life, it is not so much a question of us weaving our story, but of our story weaving us.

Consider that statement again: In life, it is not so much a question of us weaving our story, but of our story weaving us. This suggestion is very difficult to accept because it is counter-intuitive. It is not how we subjectively experience life. But consider this: Are you having these thoughts or are these thoughts having you?

Theatre is a corollary of the mind. And how we experience theatre is a reflection of how we experience our minds. In the theatre the story has already been decided. And the information presented, which is the story being told, is being presented after that fact. However, we experience theatre in the present tense, which is to say, as the subjective experience of a story unfolding. Our minds suspend their disbelief to deny the fact of the matter: that the story in front of us has already been determined. And so our minds willingly collude in the artifice. This is a reflection of our subjective experience of life, where we intuitively believe that we are in control of our own story and constantly making up our minds.

Over two thousand years ago, the Greek philosopher Aristotle wrote *Poetics.* It is the earliest surviving work of dramatic theory. In it he articulates and examines what have become the first principles of Western drama. And he offers an analysis of successful drama, concluding that plot, by which he means, story, is the single most important element of drama and that good plots follow the cause and effect of an event or action in a plausible, yet surprising, manner.

From before Aristotle's codification of drama to the present day, the theatre has reflected the mind's urge to narrative. And we will always enjoy plausible and surprising stories because it is through stories that we subjectively experience and consciously explain life. And so we feel the formula to be right. Understanding why we assume the formula to be right can assist us in our daily lives by helping us to understand and perhaps even challenge the stories our minds tell us about our selves. It can also assist theatre-makers in their telling of their tall tales. Furthermore, understanding the mind's urge to narrative and the intuitive story telling that theatre reflects, offers theatre-makers the opportunity to challenge their own minds and their chosen art form. And so in turn broaden the opportunities and challenges that the theatre can offer us, the audience.

We are not in control of our own story. Just as in the theatre, the story in front of us has already been determined. At this moment, we are the latest version of the story our mind is telling us. And this story is powerful. We find it extremely difficult to challenge, let alone change. Imagine a Pentecostalist attempting to change an Islamist's mind. Remember the last time you were in an argument, when someone else attempted to change your mind.

The unsettling truth is that we do not have the free will that we think we have. However, this does not mean that we are just deluded zombies, completely subject to the laws of determinism. Our minds have the precious ability to interrupt the story they are telling us. We do not have free will, but we do have free wont. I find myself walking outside and putting a cigarette in my mouth. As I'm about to light it: 'What's the story?' 'You want a cigarette.' 'Hold on.' And so

I interrupt the story and thereby give myself the opportunity of changing the story.

Free wont is our opportunity to change our own story. It works by giving us a thinking space. A space where we can consciously consider and judge the story our mind is telling us about a behaviour, a thought, a feeling. And this in turn gives us the opportunity to challenge the story being told, and so the potential to change it. In normal life, exercising free wont and taking the thinking space it offers is difficult. This is because in normal life we are active and so our minds consider us to be in potential danger. Our minds therefore intuitively discourage change and its prerequisite, thought, preferring to repeat today the behaviour, thoughts and feelings that allowed us to survive yesterday. This is why our habits and our beliefs prove so stubborn when challenged.

Theatre offers us a safe thinking space. In the theatre we, the audience, are not actors. And so our minds intuit no danger from the alternative actions, thoughts and feelings being presented. After all, the imagined actions, thoughts and feelings in front of us are not real and they and their consequences are not ours to negotiate. And so the mind feels safe from the threat of change.

This is often cited as the great weakness of theatre: That theatre does not lead to action or change in the real lives of its audience because theatre does not directly affect the real lives of its audience. The opposite is true. It is precisely *because* theatre does not directly affect our normal lives that our minds allow us the thinking space to experience and consider the alternative stories and behaviours in front of us.

We are safer in the theatre than in our normal lives for a second reason. Our brains are hard-wired to learn and to promote survival. But they are also hard-wired to be pleasure seekers. Our brains deliver thoughts, feelings and actions, which encourage safety, which is to say, repetition. But in the mix, they also deliver exciting and disturbing desires both in unconscious action and in intrusive fantasy. Consciousness can assist survival when the brain's demand for pleasurable over-indulgence or random waywardness becomes threatening, by relegating such ideas. But in so doing our minds deny a huge part of our potential for change.

In the safety of the theatre our minds are released from their survival instinct. And so in the theatre our minds can be radicals. Again, it is precisely because our experience of theatre does not have to lead to action or change in our normal lives that our minds have a wonderful freedom. And in this way, theatre offers our minds the opportunity to safely consider the creative possibilities of deviance. And so to safely consider our potential waywardness as opportunity rather than threat. This is why theatre is the art form of the potential of the human mind. And the potential of our mind to change.

In this century, neuroscientists and neuropsychologists are asking the most remarkable and demanding questions about what it means to be human. Neuroscience is the study of the brain and the central nervous system. Neuropsychology is the study of the relationship between behaviour, emotion and cognition on the one hand and brain function on the other. And the contemporary theatre has something to learn from both.

The essays which follow consider a few of the remarkable questions that neuroscience and neuropsychology are currently exploring. They are offered to the reader as thinking spaces and to contemporary theatre-makers as explanations for our continued use of Aristotle's codification of theatre. The final essay is a provocation and asks how we can challenge and use the codifications that theatre so intuitively relies upon. Medicine is inspired by damage and deficits. Theatre is inspired by hope and potential. And it is the hope of this volume to inspire a reconsideration of the potential of theatre, in its continuing exploration of the possibilities of being human.

1. The Urge to Narrative

I'M IN A theatre. The lights go down. Silence. I'm in the dark. Nothing. I hear music. Information. And *immediately* my mind starts trying to ruin its evening. 'What's the story? What's the story?' 'The music is sad.' Says my mind. 'It's going to be a sad story. It's old music. Sort of Russian-ish. It's going to be a sad old story set in Russia.' Lights slowly illuminate an artificial setting; a deteriorating house and veranda in a garden. 'What's the story?' Demands my brain. 'Deteriorating house and veranda. Definitely a sad story, old, probably Russian, about things deteriorating. The lights are coming up slowly. So a sad, old, probably Russian story which is going to be told slowly.' Lights illuminate a person; an old woman, sitting, knitting. 'What's the story?' 'She's not the protagonist, she's too old. And heroes don't knit. Where's the hero?' Another person enters. A younger man. 'He might be the hero. He's not knitting.' The younger man is wearing a cream suit. 'He's wearing white, well not white, but he's definitely not wearing black so he looks more like a goody than a baddy, so maybe he is the hero…' And so my mind continues, furiously interpreting the information presented and in so doing inadvertently sabotaging its own evening.

Our minds can't help themselves in their issuing of explanations. And this is because our brains are hard-wired to confabulate, which is to say, to story-tell. In the late 1940's the Japanese Canadian neurologist, Juhn Wada, developed a test to determine which side of the brain controlled speech. Today the test is used prior to brain surgery in order to determine which side of the patient's brain is responsible for key cognitive functions, and it involves injecting a drug into one hemisphere of the brain at a time. The effect is to shut down language and, or memory function in that hemisphere in order to evaluate the other half of the brain. Once the drug has been administered the patient is engaged in a series of tests or prompts. Memory, for example, is tested by showing the patient a series of pictures. And then within a few minutes, as soon as the effect of the drug has worn off, the ability to recall is tested. Wada tests are crucial as they reveal significant differences between patients, but one interesting generalisation that they have revealed is that the left hemisphere of the human brain is responsible for linear reasoning and language. So a common occurrence is for a prompt that has been made to a patient's awake right hemisphere (for example, during the test a neurologist has instructed the patient to laugh) to be subsequently explained by the patient's awake left hemisphere as a comprehensible and palatable action ('I laughed because of the amusing comment you made'). The Wada test confirms the left hemisphere as our confabulator, our spin-doctor, continually editing and presenting plausible and tolerable explanations for our behaviour. The fact is, we cannot help but tell ourselves stories because we are story-telling machines.

The stories we tell ourselves follow specific patterns. Essentially one pattern dominates, the inference equation of effect therefore cause: That happened because…; She did that because…; I feel this because…; I think this because… and so on. But the inference equation that operates is choosy, in that the explanations our minds look for, offer and accept must seem credible and probable to a given context or social world. Aristotle's insistence that successful theatre stories follow a plausible cause and effect formula within the world of a given performance articulates this invisible pattern that dominates and underpins the way our minds operate. And although our minds will readily skew explanations to justify our own behaviour, thoughts and feelings they insist in doing so within this pattern. This is also why we feel so irritated if the theatre exposes us to a story or character that does not follow the plausible cause and effect schema, and why our minds feel able to dismiss the lie of the story being told as 'unbelievable'.

A second obvious pattern operates when we are exposed to stories, again described by Aristotle. This is the governing story formula of beginning, middle and end. It is such an intuitively obvious conception that it is worth considering why this should be so. The psychoanalysist Bruno Bettelheim saw the beginning, middle, end paradigm as a consequence of the comforting bedtime stories we were told as children. Safe stories, he believed, begin with a clear premise (usually by introducing a hero and then presenting him with a difficult challenge), develop in an exciting manor (usually by placing the hero in jeopardy), and have a satisfying resolution (usually involving the triumph of the hero) in order to help us sleep. In other words, such a pattern unconsciously reassures us that there is some underlying order to our chaotic and frightening lives.

The beginning, middle, end paradigm is how our minds consider potential action in the face of threat. Our left-brain spin-doctor begins with one of two clear premises: Either: I face a challenge because I want something or I face a challenge because of an event. It then imaginatively considers a development: I could act in order to get what I want or I could act in this way or that to cope with the event. It assumes that all action leads to danger, either excitement or jeopardy. And because its evolutionary goal is its own safety it speculates on how to resolve potential consequent dramas caused by its potential action. This process is largely unconscious. And because our minds assume that all action is dangerous they tend towards self-conservation, which means our minds tend to inhibit behaviour in order to keep itself safe. This explains the enduring use of Dutch courage in human courtship, alcohol being the great disinhibitor.

The dominant story paradigm is used by our minds to justify inaction and to consider the opportunity of action. This explains why there are only three possible endings to any individual narrative: the sad ending, where the hero is thwarted (confirmation of the safety of inaction); the happy ending, where the hero gets what he wants (the opportunity of action); and the unexpected ending, where the hero is neither happy nor sad because he is surprised, having learned or achieved something unanticipated (both the threat and opportunity of action). And because the stories that our minds tell are to do with its own survival and development they are either about getting what we want (where the hero initiates) or coping with the challenges life throws at us (where the hero responds) or a mixture of the two.

Our minds have an urge to narrative and more specifically, narrative patterns. This is because our minds construct the world by using narrative patterns and interpret the world and the people in it by pattern seeking. Narrative reflects our minds' mode of understanding events and actions. And the narrative patterns our minds use follow a specific schema. This is why all stories share a similar architecture and why our minds are well equipped to sabotage their evening in the theatre because they unconsciously assume that stories must follow a logic based on an explanatory inference equation of effect therefore cause within a governing story formula of beginning, middle and end. As soon as the mind suspects the narrative engine of a story has begun, either in life or in the theatre, it will judge the plausibility of the story by this pattern. And the mind recognises that a story has begun as soon as it has identified the person whose action will most plausibly initiate the story paradigm or whose active response the story paradigm demands. In the theatre this person is called the protagonist.

2. *The 'I'*

IN A WONDERFUL euphemism, the cognitive scientist and philosopher David Chalmers calls it *the hard problem*: how do physical processes in our brains give rise to subjective experience? Or to put it another way: how does the kilo and a half of meat that is our brain become our mind? It is perhaps the greatest scientific and philosophic riddle of all.

Neuropsychologically, the self is a fiction. If you look into an open head and watch a surgeon tug and probe, you understand with a sudden and extremely shocking conviction that there's nothing more to it. There's nobody there. There's nobody home. Neurologically, our life is just a bundle of interconnected sensations and thoughts and the mental processes underlying our sense of self, our thoughts, feelings and memories are scattered through different zones of the brain. There is no special point of convergence, no experiencer of our experiences working the controls, no ego guiding our body through the world, no central core; no essence, no ego, no I.

However, the idea that there is no 'I' beyond the 'I' of grammar is very, very difficult for us to accept. And this is because it is *not* how our minds experience life. We experience life through an intuitive, subjective assumption: as an 'I', as a person with an essential being that distinguishes us from others, especially when we are considering ourselves introspectively.

Our experience of theatre is a corollary of our subjective experience of ourselves. And in theatre, we experience drama by watching the thoughts, feelings and actions of what we willingly misinterpret to be essential beings, coming into conflict with other essential beings and with what we take to be their essential inner selves.

In our subjective lives we experience ourselves as protagonists. The word protagonist is derived from the Greek, *protagonistes,* which means 'the one who plays the first part' or 'chief actor'. The protagonist will either be responsible for initiating the story or responding to the story. And this is why, in the theatre, we the audience will always identify most readily with the chief actor. Because within the context of the theatre story the protagonist is a mirror of our intuitive sense of our selves within the context of the story of our lives.

Dramatists and theatre-makers have used the device of the protagonist for over two thousand years. And Aristotle's codification of successful drama as being a good story that subjects a protagonist to a sudden, traumatic change is still the formula most used in theatre. It works like this: The protagonist is either content or discontent. If he is content then he will suffer a change in his physical, social or mental world. If he is discontent then he will effect a change. The change starts the narrative engine, or story, of the drama. Thus begun, the story continues as we experience the protagonist either becoming reconciled to, attempting to challenge or achieving change. And the drama concludes once reconciliation, challenge or achievement is complete.

The premise on which every theatrical protagonist is built is a corollary of our intuitive, subjective sense of our self; that we are an essential 'I'. And because the narrative engine of drama is a corollary of how we subjectively experience life: Change – reconciliation, challenge or achievement – leading to another change – leading to another reconciliation, challenge or achievement and so on; we the audience unconsciously accept the protagonist-traumatic change formula and will follow a hero on any trials and tribulations he may face, however fantastical, so long as they seem plausible within the context of his world. Furthermore, the experience of a protagonist and the story in which he finds himself, will be most satisfying to our minds if it presents a corollary of our minds' intuitive assumption that change is dangerous.

An old theatrical adage would have it that there is no such thing as small parts, only small actors. This is clearly nonsense and yet at the same time it is true when the theatre-maker understands that all characters, however small, have to follow the same formula as that of the protagonist. And for our minds to be satisfied with any character they must follow a story with its own beginning, middle and end in relationship to the dominant story of the protagonist. In the theatre, Shakespeare is the greatest example of this knowledge at work. Shakespeare's protagonists tended to be Kings. This is theatrically useful as the actions of Kings have immediate implications for the Kings' subjects, i.e. everybody else. And so a change initiated or suffered by one of his protagonists, set in motion the same formula for every other character. And once this formula is set in motion, within a specific narrative pattern, our minds are free to enjoy the difficulties and achievements of every other 'I' as they think, feel and act in response.

3. *Emotion, Thought and Action*

'THERE IS NOTHING either good or bad but thinking makes it so.' Shakespeare's profound insight into the nature of the relationship between human thought and emotion anticipates the development of Cognitive Behavioural Therapy by nearly four centuries. Cognitive Behavioural Therapy presents human psychology as a triangular relationship of thought, action and feeling in dynamic interaction to situation. And it emphasises the value of thought in challenging and changing unhelpful thought-action-feeling patterns, which can arise within, and disturb, an individual. The way we think about things, the way we interpret our thoughts, determines how we feel and behave. It is such a simple idea that we rarely appreciate its importance, that if we take a space to consciously reflect on the unconscious patterns we live by then we give ourselves a great gift, the opportunity to change.

Everything in the theatre is underpinned by action. Action is what motivates stories and allows emotions and thoughts to occur. An actor is a person who acts. And in the theatre actors will intuitively search for what it is they want to achieve in a particular scene or in a particular encounter. 'What is my action?' They will ask. In order to act an actor's mind needs to know its objective. And in watching theatre, an audience's mind will search for the objectives of each character and wait for them to be complete. Only after the fact of action will an actor or an audience accept emotion and thought as legitimate. And in this, once again, our experience of theatre is a corollary of our experience of our own minds.

In the 1980s the physiologist Benjamin Libit conducted a series of experiments that demonstrated that unconscious electrical processes in the brain precede conscious decisions to perform an action. Since the 1960s it had been know that voluntary motor actions are preceded in the brain by a *readiness potential*. Readiness potential is a shift in the brain's electrical potential that can be recorded by electrodes on a subject's scalp. And it occurs up to a second or more before a given action takes place. Libet's contribution was to measure a third moment as well as the start of the action and the start of the brain's readiness potential. He also measured the start of the conscious decision to act. And his results showed that conscious decision occurs just under half a second after readiness potential. Half a second is a very long time in terms of neurological activity and Libit's findings are still considered to be controversial as they imply that unconscious processes cause volitional acts which are then retrospectively felt to be consciously motivated by the subject. This of course has huge implications for the fundamental assumption we live by: the idea that we have free will. Libit himself thought that we do have free will, just not the kind of free will we assume. He noted that consciousness has the power to veto action. In other words, that we do not have free will, but we do have free wont.

The neuroscientist Michael Gazzaniga studies patients that have undergone split-brain surgery. His patients tend to be epileptics who have had corpus callostomies. The corpus callosum is the structure in the brain that facilitates communication between its two hemispheres and corpus callostomies are brain operations in which the corpus callosum is cut, thereby preventing one hemisphere from communicating with the other. The goal in such surgery is to prevent epileptic seizures spreading from one hemisphere to another. Like Libit before him, Gazzaniga discovered that the brain's two hemispheres process information differently and can therefore come to different conclusions about what should be done in response to the information before it. He devised an apparatus that flashed words on a screen at which split-brain subjects were staring. Words were flashed on the left side of the screen and which would therefore register only on the right hemisphere of a subject's brain (because our optic nerves 'cross' on their way to the brain) and words flashed on the right side of the screen, which would register only in the left hemisphere. Gazzaniga found that when the right hemisphere was presented with a prompt word like 'wave' a patient would automatically perform the action; and when later asked why he did so, the patient would rationalise his behaviour and claim to have seen someone he knew. The disturbing conclusion of Gazzaniga's research is that we routinely do not know why we do what we do because so much of our behaviour is caused by brain systems that operate without our conscious knowledge.

These findings and arguments are neither controversial nor disturbing in the theatre.

Theatre is a corollary of the mind, and its narrative architecture of stories and plots assumes that action occurs first, and the conscious awareness of feeling and thought second. Stories begin with the action of, or an event that demands action from, the protagonist. And for our minds to accept a story, as plausible, these actions must be retrospectively understandable by the inference equation: effect (action) *therefore* cause (plausible explanation). In the theatre our minds assume that action precedes conscious thought and emotion. Because our minds intuit that without action there will be very little to feel or think about. So in theatre, it is only once action begins that our minds will allow themselves to enjoy the relationship between thought, emotion and potential future action manifested in the characters.

We all strive for cognitive coherence in our lives. Cognitive therapies tend to deal with people suffering *cognitive dissonance*. The idea is this: Cognitive dissonance arises whenever an individual simultaneously holds two psychologically inconsistent cognitions ('I love X but am falling in love with Y'). And because dissonance induces psychological discomfort or tension, it drives the individual to seek consonance. Our minds do this automatically and this is the reason why we will always first justify our behaviour in the face of challenge ('X has many faults that I've tolerated for far too long; I have every right to be falling in love with Y' or, 'I'm no good for X, she would be better off without me'). In the theatre our minds enjoy experiencing the cognitive dissonance of the characters in front of them. More than this, our minds *expect* to see cognitive dissonance being played out and will feel cheated if this does not happen. And our minds assume from the theatre what they find so difficult to admit in real life: that it is unconscious emotion and not conscious thought that tends to form our beliefs and motivate our actions.

The neuropsychologist Paul Broks demonstrates the primacy of emotion in decision-making by considering disgust. He suggests two demonstrative scenarios. Scenario one: a man goes to the supermarket and buys an oven-ready chicken. Gets it home, slips on a condom, and has sex with it. And then he cooks it and serves it to his friends for dinner. Why, he asks, do we think this is wrong? No one is any the wiser. The meat is uncontaminated and everyone enjoyed their meal. Scenario two: one day, after a nice chicken dinner, our friend and his sister decide they would like to have sex together. Just the *once*. So they do. Enjoyably. Using contraception, and agreeing to keep it a secret. It's a beautiful, one-off experience that enhances their relationship. So why do we think *this* is wrong? No one got hurt. The fact is, most people can't give a convincing reason. They are morally dumbfounded – believing intuitively that something is wrong but being stuck for a rational justification. The reason we feel like this is because we think that we use reason to make moral judgments, when actually it is our emotions that guide us. In the theatre our minds take this for granted and they search for the strongest motivating emotion in every character, and they *expect* it to cause dissonance either within a character or between characters.

The opportunity of the theatre is to offer our minds a thinking space, because conscious thought can change thoughts, feelings and actions. But our minds will only accept the legitimacy of the theatre and therefore its opportunity, if the narrative before it demonstrates its own workings, which is to say: that action occurs before conscious thought and emotion and that in the conflict between unconscious emotion and thought, emotion is our dominant motivator. And because it is emotion that leads us to our moral conclusions, our minds will intuitively identify with any character attempting to achieve something that they *feel* to be right and intuitively reject any character attempting to achieve something that they *feel* to be wrong.

4. Empathy

WE ARE BORN with emotional impulses which draw us to others. And our minds are hard-wired to connect with those around us and to resonate with them. This is why a day old baby will cry when it hears another baby cry. Empathy is a development of this rudimentary impulse. It is the ability to imagine the psychological and emotional circumstances of another. And it enables us to imagine how our own behaviour might affect others. Empathy, therefore, allows us to sympathise with, and to understand others, by imaginatively putting ourselves in another's psychological, emotional shoes. And this in turn enables us to deliberately inflict either kindness or hurt on others by allowing us to imaginatively concoct specifically intentioned behaviour.

Our emotions tend to arouse matching emotions. Such a response has a huge survival value. If others are showing fear or distress there may be a very good reason for you to be worried too. And so we intuitively mimic the emotions and behaviour of others. We do this especially with the emotions and behaviour of people we like. And this is why pick-up artists and other con men use mimicry in their courting of targets, because they know that being with someone who adopts deviating body postures results in fewer good feelings about them than being with someone who dutifully copies every move the other makes.

Empathy is activated by the emotional presence, physical behaviour and story of another rather than by any objective evaluation. The mechanisms by which empathy works are most easily explained by studying people who do not have it, *autists*. Autism is a brain development disorder characterized by impaired social interaction and communication, and by restricted and repetitive behavior. There are many kinds of autism but all autists share a common deficiency: they have no theory of mind.

Theory of mind is the ability to attribute mental states like beliefs, intents and desires to oneself and others based on the silent presumption that others have a mind like our own. For most of us it is intuitive, and this is why most of us take our theory of mind for granted. One of the most important milestones in theory of mind development is gaining the ability to attribute *false belief*. This means that we are able to recognize that others can have beliefs about the world that are 'wrong'. And to do this we need to understand how knowledge is formed, that people's beliefs are based on *their* knowledge, that mental states can differ from reality, and that people's behavior can be predicted by their mental states. A key test that developmental psychologists use to measure theory of mind is called the Sally-Anne Test.

Sally and Anne are dolls. Sally has a basket and Anne has a box. Experimenters show their subject a simple scene in which Sally places a marble in her basket and then leaves the room. While Sally is absent, Anne takes the marble out of Sally's basket and puts it into her box. Sally then returns and the subject is asked where they think Sally will look for her marble. The subject is said to 'pass' the test if they understand that Sally will most likely look for the marble where she left it, inside her basket. Subjects under the age of four and most autistic children of older ages 'fail' the test. They are seemingly unaware of Sally's false belief, which is to say, what Sally *does not know*, that the marble has been moved. Most of us learn, and are able, to anticipate what others know and therefore how they might behave on the basis of that knowledge. Learning that others are capable of holding false beliefs is the prerequisite to understanding that other people have different thoughts and feelings from our own. A fully developed theory of mind is what allows us to engage in our finely tuned social behaviour, because it enables us to predict the behaviour of others accurately. Autists lack this ability and this is one reason why they are sometimes called *mind-blind*.

Autists are termed mind-blind for a second reason: they cannot read faces. Most newborn babies prefer faces to any other visual stimulus. Within two days they can imitate surprised, sad and happy faces and within two weeks a child will mirror more specific movements of its mother's eyes and lips. We are hard-wired to respond to faces and hard-wired to read them. And we do this by *seeing* emotion. The psychologist Paul Ekman has shown that the facial expressions of the six basic emotions (anger, disgust, fear, joy, sadness and surprise) are universal across human cultures. And most minds are beautifully attuned to the stream of emotional signals emanating from other people's faces and postures and intuitively resonate with corresponding expressions of our own. Autists suffer both an impaired theory of mind, which means they lack an intuitive understanding that other people have minds that are separate from their own, and an impaired ability to interpret and signal facial expressions. This means that the social interactions we take for granted prove extremely complicated for them. And this is why they lack empathy, because empathy relies on an intuitive theory of mind and an unconscious ability to *see* emotion. This also explains why autists tend to be so impressively individualistic, being as they are, totally immune to peer pressure.

Empathy is morally selective and geographically and socially limited. It is triggered most strongly in children when they witness the distress of another in the face of a perceived injustice. And this is the same for audiences in the theatre. However its power diminishes when children witness a similar event in a social group different to their own, and the greater the difference in the social group, the less the empathy. This phenomenon has a solid evolutionary explanation, where an intuitive bond and sense of justice to the nurturing group was helpful for the individuals' survival within the group and in the face of competition from other groups. And this explains the origin of tribes. One of the great potentials of theatre is the fact that in the theatre, this rule does not hold.

Our minds experience the theatre as an extension of the shared imaginative play, which originally helped develop and hone our theory of mind. This is why our minds will always identify most with the person or character we like the best. And why our minds will always both empathise and sympathise most with a character suffering, or fighting, an injustice. In the theatre this will usually be the protagonist. However, in the safety of the lie that is the theatre, our minds allow themselves to empathise with, and feel for, other people. In the theatre our minds are able to *extend* their capacity for empathy and will *more readily* empathise with characters from social groups different to our own. The extended empathy which theatre elicits has two very valuable implications.

Theatre can help to sensitise us to the emotions of other people who come from, what our minds would normally consider to be, a 'competing' group. This is because our minds feel safe in the theatre, intuiting that empathy within the lie of the theatre does not have to impinge on our real lives. So the first implication of the extended empathy that our minds allow in the theatre is an increased understanding, and appreciation, of different racial, traditional, religious and social groups. The second implication of extended empathy is an increased understanding of the social implications of our emotions. For example, in ordinary life when we are sexually attracted to someone, we tend to become solipsistic, and hostile towards those we perceive to be potential rivals. In the theatre we not only feel for the character in love, but we also feel for the other characters as well. Which means that in the theatre we can both feel emotion *and* understand its social implications without our usual, self-interested, involvement. And so the theatre can help us to both refine and broaden our human and humane capacities of emotional understanding. And this is why the stories theatre tells and the characters it invites us to empathize with, will only truly satisfy our minds if they in some way demonstrate the benefits and complications of human morality.

5. *Morality*

THROUGH THE ENJOYABLE distractions of story (what happens), plot (how the story happens) and character (who the story happens to) all theatre explores a theme: what the piece of theatre is actually about. In theatre, the theme is the hidden unifying idea. And it is perplexing to notice that when the theme is made effable, which means, when the theme of a piece of theatre is directly articulated, our minds become annoyed by, and blocked to, the exploration unfolding in front of them. In the best theatre, story, plot and character, as well as following plausible mind paradigms of their own, also serve as *functions* of the theme being explored.

There are a limitless number of themes. However the theme of a piece of theatre is as much a lie as its story, plot and characters; which is to say, the theme is merely a territory; a defined linguistic landscape, to allows the true exploration of all theatre: the potential of human being-ness in the face of human desire. In great theatre works, which are plays that prove continually fascinating to successive generations, the theme *is* a desire. But all theatre is fundamentally an exploration of human desire, explored through the language of a theme, and using a story which promotes a central conflict between a protagonist whose function is to demonstrate the positive aspect of human desire and an antagonist whose function is to demonstrate its negative aspect.

Theatre is a corollary of the mind and the theme being explored is a lexicon, which allows the presentation of our minds' desire. Desire is a sense of longing for a person, object or outcome. And the satisfaction of a desire usually involves pleasure. Desire is innate and is helpful to sustaining life because it promotes pleasurable action like eating, care giving and of course sex. And the lack of desire, though often cited as the *true* potential of human being-ness, usually results not in absolute contentment but in a perplexing and frustrating state which we have all experienced: boredom. Our minds value and rationalise our desires but they also intuit that desire, when unmitigated, is dangerous to life. And this is because extreme desire tends to generate extreme action, which in turn tends to generate conflict. And so our minds have an ambivalent relationship to their own desires, both recognising that the choices we typically make depend on our desires while at the same time devoting vast quantities of conscious energy attempting to mitigate our extreme desires. This is why we feel less dissonance when conforming to accepted standards of social or professional behaviour and why we place so much store by our intuitive sense of right and wrong. This helps explain the golden rule that underpins the world's great religions: do unto others as you would have done onto you. And it suggests that our minds are hard-wired to be moral.

The evolutionary biologist Marc Hauser has conducted a study into the nature of moral judgments called: The Moral Sense Test. In the test participants from all over the world were presented with a series of hypothetical moral dilemmas and asked to judge each one. One dilemma introduces Oscar, taking his daily walk near some train tracks and suddenly noticing that the approaching train is out of control. Oscar can see what has happened: the driver of the train saw five men walking across the tracks and slammed on the brakes, but the brakes failed and the driver fainted. The train is now rushing toward the five men and is moving so fast that they will not be able to get off the track in time. Fortunately, Oscar is standing next to a switch that will temporarily turn the train onto a side track. There is a heavy object on the side track and if the train hits the object, the object will slow the train down, thereby giving the men time to escape. Unfortunately, there is a man standing on the side track in front of the heavy object, with his back turned. Oscar's dilemma is simple: he can throw the switch, preventing the train from killing the men, but in so doing it will kill the man. Or he can refrain from doing this, letting the five die. So: is it morally permissible for Oscar to throw the switch? The amazing result of Hauser's test was that every participant, no matter where they were from in the world, responded in exactly the same way. They all decided that Oscar must throw the switch. The only differences occurred in interpretation. This suggests that although the way our minds express their decision making is culturally determined, most human minds have a hard-wired and universally similar, moral architecture.

Our minds intuitively recognise the fact that we are a bundle of competing impulses, which attempt to motivate us in different directions and they rely on their inbuilt moral sense to determine action. In the theatre this reality is given expression by competing characters who personify the different conscious and unconscious 'voices' competing for control over our thoughts feelings and actions and which are prompted by innate desires. And our minds will feel most satisfied in the theatre if the story comes to a moral conclusion, which confirms that extreme desire is dangerous. This is why one of our favoured characters in the theatre is the psychopath. Psychopathy is a personality disorder whose hallmark is a lack of empathy. And the psychopath's function in the theatre in terms of the theme is to demonstrate the danger of untempered desire. So in the mind of the psychopath, which is to say, in the part of our mind that is psychopathic, love becomes lust, power becomes paranoia, justice becomes revenge and self-knowledge becomes justification. And because our minds are intuitively moral, they will enjoy seeing the psychopath receiving his just desserts and they will feel terribly unsettled if he does not. In the safety of the theatre our minds will be most satisfied if they can have their cake and eat it, which is to say, if the theatre both plays out extreme desires while at the same time, confirming their danger.

In 1971 a team of researchers led by the psychologist Philip Zimbardo conducted the now infamous Stanford Prison Experiment. The experiment was conceived to explore the psychological effects of social roles within a given social environment. And it made use of a prisoner, prison guard scenario. Twenty-four undergraduates were selected to play the roles of both guards and prisoners and live in a mock prison in the basement of the Stanford psychology building. Those selected were chosen for their lack of psychological issues, crime history, and medical disabilities, in order to obtain a representative sample. Roles were assigned based on a coin toss. The results of the experiment were shocking. Not only did the students adapt easily to their assigned roles, but they quickly stepped far beyond the boundaries of what had been predicted. One-third of the 'guards' were judged to have exhibited genuine sadistic tendencies, while many of the 'prisoners' were emotionally traumatized. Zimbardo concluded that both prisoners and guards had become too grossly absorbed in their roles and terminated the experiment after six days. The results have a profound implication for our moral minds because they suggest that situation can influence our behaviour more than our inherent individual personality.

Our minds experience the theatre as an extension of the shared imaginative play, which originally helped develop and hone our theory of mind. And the implication of the Stanford Prison Experiment reveals another possibility of theatre to help us develop our more humane capacities. In life, our minds are less aware of the social world they inhabit, and social role it plays, tending to take both for granted. In the theatre it *sees* the social world in front of it and so is able to judge its impact on character. And this is why Shakespeare intuitively counterpointed three environments: the world of the court which is an environment that promotes politics in the pursuit of survival and power and therefore allows an examination of actions based on extreme thought; the worlds of the street or tangled forest which promote the appetites in pursuit of pleasure and therefore allows an examination of actions based on extreme emotion; and the world of the countryside where thought, emotion and action are held in a naturally open balance. So by presenting characters that personify the many competing voices within our mind, in relation to a motivating theme, and subject to a dominant environment, the theatre can offer us a tool in the management of our desires. And it can therefore assist in the maturing of our intuitive, but susceptible, moral minds.

6. *Transcendence*

OUR MINDS HAVE a sense that there is something above and beyond material existence. A hunch that reality's visible, tangible, sensual face, which we savour and appreciate with our five senses, is not all. They have an impulse that there is an invisible reality that animates, and yet goes beyond, the visible. Many thinkers worry at the discussion of transcendence, as in our minds it seems bound to our idea of the numinous, which is to say, our idea of the divine. But let us not worry, let us explore.

Our minds have the capacity to hold rational thoughts alongside irrational intuitions. This is why we can experience theatre; knowing that what is in front of us is a fabrication while at the same time investing it with emotional integrity. Magical thinking infuses our lives: we cross our fingers, knock on wood and refuse to walk under ladders. Even if we deny belief in the supernatural we are all inclined towards magical thinking and its cousin, superstition. We may not believe in ghosts but would still rather not pitch our tents in a graveyard. Magical thinking is the source of our creativity, our dream worlds and our imaginations. And it is universal: every culture has its own folklore, myths, fairytales, religion and theatre. But transcendence is more than magical thinking.

Distinguishing memories of events that really happened from events we have only imagined is difficult. And suggests that the sharp line we tend to draw between reality and imagination is, in fact, porous. An extreme example of this is Korsakoff's syndrome, a brain disorder caused by a lack of vitamin B, where sufferers characteristically guess an answer to a question or imagine an event and then mistake their guess or imagination for an actual memory. This tendency is called confabulation; *with fable.* Less extreme examples include psychosomatic illnesses. Common experiences involve confusing a dressing gown for a person, or a discarded pullover for a cat. And the reality is that we all have a tendency to confabulate. In a now classic experiment the psychologist Cheves Perky asked 'normal' subjects to look at a blank screen and to imagine an object on it, like a tomato. Unbeknownst to the subjects she back-projected a picture of a tomato onto the screen, gradually increasing its brightness. Even when the picture was bright enough to be easily seen, the subjects still believed that they were imagining it. It is clear that the difference between our objective and subjective worlds can be imprecise. And this is why the legal profession places little store by uncorroborated evidence. However, transcendence is more than just the perforations between our imaginary and real thoughts.

The idea of transcendence somehow relates to what Albert Einstein described as the source of all true science, the most beautiful and profound experience that is the sensation of the mystical. The psychologist and philosopher William James proposed four marks that justify calling an experience mystical. They are: ineffability (that the *experience* somehow defies description in words), noetic (a term he coined to describe the idea of knowingness through illumination), transiency (as such experiences are temporary in nature), and passivity (because such experiences can not be induced to order and once they begin the feeling is of ones own will being in abeyance).

The ultimate aim of theatre is to create a corollary of our sense of transcendence. In the theatre, unlike in life, the conditions, which can generate such an experience, can be constructed. And it will always be a single moment where story, plot, character and theme coincide in an intense and pure communication of what our minds understand as a deeply intuited knowledge. The experience of transcendence somehow defies words. And in the theatre it is located in a transforming action; the meeting of the small and the monumental within the actor, which both distils the entire experience of the theatrical event and yet somehow manages to go beyond it. In Shakespeare's *Measure for Measure* it is found in the decision moment before Isabella kneels to save her brother, in *King Lear* it is located in Lear's entrance, carrying the dead Cordelia in his arms; in Bertolt Brecht's *Mother Courage* it is the single Mother once again taking up her wagon; in Samuel Beckett's *Waiting for Godot* it is in Vladimir and Estragon's 'not moving' after they decide to go; in Arthur Miller's *The Crucible* it is located in Proctor's tearing of his confession; in Brian Friel's *Dancing at Lughnasa* it breaks through in the sisters' dance. The quality of these moments depends on the talents of the ensemble presenting the whole, but they are there and they remain the most profound communications *within* these great works.

In a great theatre work our minds experience these moments as somehow inevitable; as if they have awakened an already existent knowledge within us. And they carry with them a curious and lasting sense of authority. They represent the most mature expression of the commonwealth of imagination, which links us all in our response to stories. Just as when a group of five year olds are told a story and we hear the same oohs and ahhs at the same moments, so these moments fuse us all. The feeling, of course, passes. And this is because; the intensity of the experience cannot survive the intrusion of thought. And these moments are for the audience and not for the actor, as they both require and feel like passivity, which is to say that we feel the experience as happening through us rather than activated by us. This is why many actors leave the stage bewildered that they have felt nothing during the performance while their audience has clearly been deeply affected by it.

The hard problem for neuroscience is to explain how physical processes in the brain give rise to subjective experience. The hard problem for theatre is achieving the corollary of transcendence. It relies on the talent of the creative ensemble and the complete success of each of the theatre's component parts: story, plot, character and theme. Theatre makers know that their attempt to manufacture such a moment can only be tested in one environment: the performance. It is only the intensity generated by placing a work in front of an audience that can yield the required focus from the actors. And it is only the passive minds of an audience that have the potential to experience such a moment.

Our minds intuitively recognise that the state of transcendence is possible in human life, and that a glimpse of this state is achievable in theatre. In both experiences our mind's own confabulation briefly ceases. And in the theatre this gives rise to a pure state of companionship; of being alone, beside another, where we sense an absolute truth: that we are each completely singular and yet at the same time completely connected by something essential. Deep within us all lays the hope that this moment will occur. This is why we *really* go to the theatre. And this explains why audiences all over the world are unanimous in their recognition of a great theatre work and damning if the theatre in front of them is only just very good.

7. *The Challenge*

HOW CAN THEATRE serve us? This is the most difficult question a theatre-maker can ask, as it contains within it an infuriating notion of the didactic. And the theatre does not serve us well when it is being didactic. The filmmaker Wim Wenders once noted that when people think that they've seen enough of something, but there's more, and no change of shot, then they react in a curiously livid way. The same response occurs in the theatre when our minds feel that in some way they are being educated.

Our minds are bundles of expectations, preferences and ways of inference geared to the greatest possible cognitive result for the smallest possible processing effort. They are able to leap to complex conclusions from the slightest information. In life they are capable of weighing up, and responding to, potential emergency in milliseconds. In the theatre they are capable of deciphering the information before them at the same speed. And our minds do this by following narrative patterns. They have evolved to use narratives because of the survival and reproductive advantages it offers. And they are particularly interested in narratives, which reflect their own subjective experience of life as a protagonist, following an emotional journey in relation to actions and events, which are then retrospectively justified or judged by thought. They are also agile social guides, hard-wired to interpret themselves and others both through outer expressions and actions and through inner thoughts and emotions. They are automatic empathisers, with their own highly developed theory of themselves, which allows an understanding of another's intentions, goals, desires and beliefs. They are intuitive moralists, preferring heroes to triumph and villains to get their just desserts. And they have a deep intuition of the transcendent, of a some-ineffable-thing, which binds us together as human beings.

Theatre is a corollary of our mind. It is our minds' invention and reflection. And the narrative patterns, which the theatre imaginatively employs, precisely reflect the patterns our minds use to explain us to ourselves. The theatre uses representative characters who mirror the mind's conception of itself as a protagonist, as an 'I'.

And it places them in complicated social situations, which exercise our minds' dual preoccupations of monitoring itself and others through its own theory of mind. The theatre specifically reflects the minds ambiguous relationship to its own internal desires in the face of its in-built moral instinct. And the theatre recognises the mind's dilemma of the primacy and danger of action. More than all of this, the theatre searches for echoes of the minds intuition of the transcendent and in so doing offers our moral minds a deep confirmation that all human life and experience is somehow connected.

Theatre does serve us *and* our minds do need education. Our minds are susceptible to the normalising and polluting effects of environments. And environments imperceptibly influence our intuitive moral compass. Moreover, our minds are sneaky. They will resolve their cognitive dissonances to suit themselves, by justifying behaviour, emotion and thought through the explanatory narratives they find most pleasurable. When we begin to understand how our minds work we can use that understanding to challenge our minds conception of themselves. The by-product of this challenge will be our ability to make better theatre. The challenge for theatre-makers, like all true challenges, is simple to articulate and difficult to achieve: to provide a better thinking space for self-reconsideration.

Conscious thought, as the cognitive behavioural therapist knows, is the gateway to change in feeling and action. Thought requires a thinking space so that an active self-reconsideration is possible. A change of thinking or a desire for behavioural change demands a conscious and sustained application of the free wont that our minds grant us. Theatre cannot help us in this, but what it can offer the mind is a thinking space. And there are two approaches theatre can take to achieve this: by confronting the mind or by cajoling it; by either directly challenging the minds conception of itself by presenting new theatrical forms or to be as furtive as our own minds and use their preferred paradigm of narrative to sneakily provoke them into thought.

Challenging the security of the mind's narrative paradigm is possible and exciting. The difficulty lies in the fact that initially our minds *will not like it*. Samuel Beckett was one of the greatest pioneers in issuing and exploring challenges to conventional theatrical forms, which is to say, conventional mind paradigms. And the critical assault, which met the premiers of his work, can be read as the minds' intuitive reaction against their usual, hard-wired thought patterns. The shock of his inventions demanded a response. For many minds the response was rejection, for a still growing number the response was to open up a thinking space. In Beckett's work form is inseparable from content. And his legacy and his preparedness to risk the mind's animosity must continue to be an inspiration for theatre-makers. In theatre, form, when scrupulously married or juxtaposed to content, can arouse reconsiderations of what it means to be human. And it requires both the courage to experiment publicly and the preparedness to risk rejection.

Using the mind's preferred narrative paradigm to reopen thought is the second option. This approach has the potential to generate a larger audience because stories, plots, characters and themes reflect the default position of our minds. And our minds will intuitively describe the echo of their own workings as the most readily satisfying theatre. Theatre-makers should be aware that by employing this paradigm that their own minds will become susceptible to the comfortable, unthinking environment of praise. The best model of the mind's preferred theatre is Shakespeare who allowed story, plot and character to exist in their own right *while* using them as functions of the theme being explored. The thinking space he promotes is in the gaps. Ancient Persian rug makers would deliberately drop a small faulty stitch into each of their creations, believing that only God could make something perfect. Shakespeare's masterpieces are likewise imperfect. In his work there are countless leaps of time that do not make sense, numerous small encounters that seem to inhibit action and repeated images that appear to overly extend speeches. Each theatre maker will decide what they feel to be extraneous for their productions, but the lesson of his work to theatre-makers is a warning against perfection. Narrative theatre is at its best when it follows the mind's paradigms, which Shakespeare so effortlessly intuited, but an unblemished play will be a closed experience. It will lead to momentary appreciation and nothing more.

Over two thousand years ago Aristotle defined what are still the first principles of Western drama. He also insisted that theatre dramatised the workings of the heart. The heart, he thought, was the source of mental life because of its dynamic action and its warmth. The brain was there to cool the blood. Two thousand years later we know this not to be true. We know that hearts can be replaced and that it is the brain that is the source of an individuals' mental life. Today, neuroscientists and neuropsychologists are asking the most remarkable and demanding questions about what it means to be human. And their discoveries not only explain why Aristotle's formulation has survived but also have a huge amount to offer contemporary theatre-makers as they consider their future work.

Our minds make us up. Not the other way around. It is our minds that consciously experience our emotions, thoughts and actions. And it is our minds that consciously consider our future emotions, thoughts and actions. Our idea of our self, of what it means to be a person and indeed what is means to be a certain type of person, is dependent on our mind. They are our storytellers, our confabulator, rationalizing and editing explanations for our feelings, thoughts and behaviours, settling on the story that seems most plausible, and offering imagined future scenarios based on that story. Theatre is a corollary of our minds. And it serves us best, when having delivered its entertainment, it also allows us a thinking space, a moment to reconsider ourselves, to ask how we can be otherwise. And the theatre can do this by either demanding a thinking space or by using the mind's own paradigms as a self-challenge.

If we believe with Socrates, that the greatest potential of the human being is 'the considered life – free, creative, informed and chosen, a life of achievement and fulfilment, of pleasure and understanding, of love and friendship; in short, the best human life in a human world, humanely lived', then the theatre can serve us best by offering us a thinking space. Which is to say, the theatre, either by demand or by slight of hand, can and does support our minds' intuitive moral sense by promoting thoughts of ethics: thinking and theorising about what is good and bad, and how people should live. Intuitively we sense that this is why our minds created theatre, and that the fact of the matter is that our mind's ambition for its creation lies beyond the curtain call. By acknowledging this, theatre-makers suddenly give themselves a realisable opportunity. For suddenly they can turn their difficult question on its head, and rather than ask: 'how can the theatre serve us?' they can ask instead: 'how can we best serve the theatre?' And we can best serve the theatre by integrating our new knowledge of the workings of the mind to help us make better work. And we can move forward with great confidence, knowing that when again the lights go down, and again we find ourselves in the dark, our minds – *all of our minds* – are deeply, silently hoping for the experience that connects each and every one of us, the experience of transcendence, which remains the most profound inspiration for our own ethical change.

The On Theatre Series

Also Available from Oberon

ON DEATH

Mick Gordon and Marie de Hennezel 978-1-84002-607-8

ON LOVE

Mick Gordon 978-1-84002-608-5

ON EGO

Mick Gordon and Paul Broks 978-1-84002-609-2

ON RELIGION: GRACE

Mick Gordon and A C Grayling 978-1-84002-797-6

ON EMOTION

Mick Gordon and Paul Broks 978-1-84002-883-6

ON EVOLUTION: THE RIDE OF YOUR LIFE

Mick Gordon 978-1-84002-958-1

ON IDENTITY: PRESSURE DROP

Mick Gordon and Billy Bragg 978-1-84002-971-0